# *The Herb Doctor's Handbook*

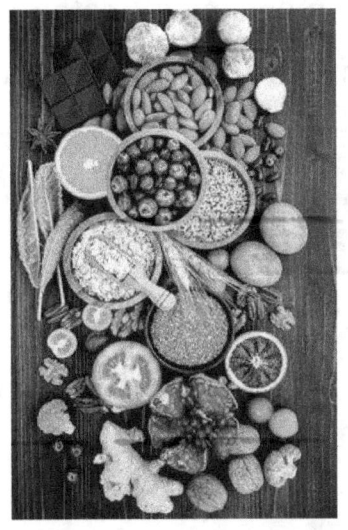

*Essential Herbs for Children's Well-being*

Dr. Sara J. Griffin

# Table Of Content

*Introduction*

*Chapter 1: Understanding Herbal Medicine for Kids*

*1.1 The History and Traditions of Herbal Healing*

*1.2 Herbal Medicine Today: Benefits and Precautions*

*1.3 Safety Considerations and Dosage Guidelines for Children*

*Chapter 2: Creating a Herbal Medicine Cabinet*

*2.1 Essential Herbs for Children's Well-being*

*2.2 Sourcing and Growing Medicinal Herbs*

*2.3 Herbal Preparation Techniques: Infusions, Tinctures, and More*

*Chapter 3: Boosting Immunity and Warding off Illness*

*3.1 Immune-Boosting Herbs and Remedies*

*3.2 Herbal Support for Common Childhood Illnesses*

*3.3 Preventive Measures: Herbs for a Healthy Immune System*

*Chapter 4: Soothing Digestive Discomforts*

*4.1 Gentle Herbs for Digestive Health*

*4.2 Herbal Remedies for Upset Stomachs and Colic*

*4.3 Supporting Healthy Digestion in Children*

*Chapter 5: Nurturing Respiratory Health*

*5.1 Herbal Allies for Respiratory Wellness*

*5.2 Managing Coughs, Colds, and Congestion with Herbs*

*5.3 Promoting Healthy Breathing in Children*

*Chapter 6: Calming the Mind and Promoting Restful Sleep*

*6.1 Herbal Solutions for Anxiety and Stress*

*6.2 Bedtime Rituals: Herbs for Peaceful Sleep*

*6.3 Supporting Healthy Emotional Well-being in Children*

*Chapter 7: Enhancing Skin Health and Healing*

*7.1 Herbal Remedies for Common Skin Issues*

*7.2 Nourishing and Soothing Herbal Skin Care*

*7.3 Herbal First Aid for Cuts, Scrapes, and Burns*

*Chapter 8: Herbal Support for Growth and Development*

*8.1 Supporting Healthy Growth with Herbs*

*8.2 Herbal Solutions for Nutritional Needs*

*8.3 Boosting Brain Power and Cognitive Function*

*Chapter 9: Integrating Herbs into Daily Life*

*9.1 Incorporating Herbs into Meals and Snacks*

*9.2 Herbal Teas, Infusions, and Tonics for Kids*

*9.3 Herbal Bathing and Body Care Rituals*

*Chapter 10: Holistic Approaches to Children's Health*

*10.1 Combining Herbs with Mind-Body Practices*

*10.2 Nature's Healing Power: Outdoor Activities and Herb Exploration*

*10.3 Cultivating a Healthy Lifestyle for Children*

*Conclusion: Empowering Parents as Herb Doctors for Their Children*

*Appendix: Quick Reference Guide to Essential Herbs and Remedies*

Glossary: Key Terms and Definitions

# Introduction

Welcome to a world where the healing power of nature meets the well-being of our little ones. In this captivating journey, we invite you to explore the realm of herbal remedies specifically designed for children's health. "The Herb Doctor's Handbook: Essential Herbs for Children's Well-being" is your key to unlocking the extraordinary potential of herbs in nurturing your child's vitality and happiness.

As parents, we strive to provide the best for our children, ensuring their health and happiness at every turn. In a world where synthetic medications and chemical-laden products dominate the market, many of us yearn for a more natural approach—a way to support our children's well-being without compromising their overall health. This is where the world of herbal remedies shines with its gentle effectiveness and time-honored wisdom.

In this book, we bridge the gap between ancient traditions and modern science, offering you a comprehensive guide to harnessing the incredible healing powers of herbs for your child's benefit. From boosting their immune system to soothing digestive discomforts, supporting respiratory health, and nurturing their emotional well-being, this handbook covers a wide spectrum of common childhood health concerns.

But "The Herb Doctor's Handbook" is not just about remedies. It's a transformative journey that empowers you, the parent or caregiver, to become an herb doctor for your child. You'll not only gain knowledge about specific herbs and their applications but also develop a deeper understanding of the principles behind herbal medicine. Armed with this knowledge, you'll be equipped to make informed decisions and tailor herbal remedies to suit your child's unique needs.

Throughout this book, you'll find practical advice, step-by-step instructions, and dosage guidelines to ensure safe and effective use of herbs. We'll guide you through creating your own herbal medicine cabinet, sourcing and growing medicinal herbs, and preparing various herbal formulations. You'll discover the art of crafting herbal teas, infusions, tinctures, and more, making it easy to incorporate herbs into your child's daily routine.

Let this journey be a testament to the power of nature's gifts and the bond between parent and child. As you delve into the pages of this handbook, you'll discover that herbs are not merely medicinal plants but compassionate allies, ready to support your child's well-being in a gentle and holistic way.

We live in a fast-paced world where it's easy to lose touch with the rhythms of nature. However, within these pages, you'll rediscover the importance of reconnecting with the natural world and incorporating its wisdom into your child's life. From cultivating herbs in a backyard garden to exploring the healing power of nature through outdoor activities, you'll find ways to infuse your child's life with the magic of plants.

"The Herb Doctor's Handbook" is not meant to replace professional medical advice. Instead, it complements and expands your understanding of children's health, providing a natural and empowering approach that aligns with your values. By combining the best of traditional wisdom and modern scientific research, we aim to equip you with the knowledge and tools to make informed choices for your child's well-being.

Throughout this book, we emphasize the importance of collaboration between parents and healthcare providers. We encourage open communication and invite you to discuss herbal remedies with your child's pediatrician or a qualified herbalist to ensure a holistic and well-rounded approach to their health.

Our intention is for "The Herb Doctor's Handbook" to be more than just a book. It's a catalyst for a transformative journey, both for you and your child. As you embrace herbal remedies, you're not only providing them with natural support but also teaching them valuable lessons about self-care, the power of nature, and the interconnectedness of mind, body, and spirit.

So, whether you're a parent, grandparent, caregiver, or simply someone passionate about nurturing children's health, this book is your invitation to embark on a remarkable adventure. Together, let's explore the wonders of herbal remedies, empower ourselves as herb doctors, and embrace a path of wellness that honors the innate wisdom of our children and the healing bounty of the earth.

Are you ready to unlock the secrets of herbal remedies and embark on this extraordinary journey? Let "The Herb Doctor's Handbook: Essential Herbs for Children's Well-being" be your guiding light as you navigate the rich tapestry of natural remedies, discover the joys of herbal medicine, and nurture your child's health with love and nature's wisdom. Let's begin this transformative chapter and embrace the world of herbs for our little ones' well-being.

# Chapter 1

# <u>Understanding Herbal Medicine for Kids</u>

## *1.1 The History and Traditions of Herbal Healing*

Throughout the ages, herbal healing has been an integral part of human civilization. Long before the advent of modern medicine, our ancestors turned to the bountiful offerings of nature to address their health concerns. The history and traditions of herbal healing are a testament to the deep-rooted connection between humans and plants, a relationship that continues to thrive today.

# 1.Ancient Civilizations and Herbal Medicine

The ancient civilizations of Egypt, China, India, and Greece hold a rich heritage of herbal medicine. These cultures recognized the healing potential of plants and developed sophisticated systems of herbal healing.

In ancient Egypt, herbal remedies were intricately woven into their religious and medical practices. Papyrus scrolls such as the Ebers Papyrus and the Edwin Smith Papyrus documented the use of herbs for various ailments and rituals.

Chinese herbal medicine, a vital component of Traditional Chinese Medicine (TCM), has a history spanning thousands of years. The Chinese developed a deep understanding of the properties and energetics of herbs and used them to restore balance and harmony within the body.

India's Ayurvedic tradition also encompasses a vast body of herbal knowledge. Ayurveda emphasizes the balance of body, mind, and spirit and utilizes herbs to restore equilibrium and promote overall well-being.

The ancient Greeks, including notable figures such as Hippocrates and Dioscorides, contributed significantly to herbal medicine. Hippocrates, often regarded as the father of Western medicine, recognized the importance of diet, lifestyle, and herbal remedies in maintaining health. Dioscorides, a Greek physician and pharmacologist, compiled the influential herbal text "De Materia Medica," which cataloged hundreds of medicinal plants.

## 2.Herbalism in Medieval Europe

During the Middle Ages, herbalism played a crucial role in healthcare practices. Monastic gardens became centers of herbal knowledge, and monks and nuns cultivated herbs for medicinal purposes. Herbalists like Hildegard von Bingen, a German Benedictine abbess, contributed valuable insights into herbal medicine through their writings and practices.

Herbs were used to treat a range of conditions, from common ailments to more complex diseases. Folk remedies and local traditions also played a significant role in shaping herbal knowledge during this period.

## 3.Indigenous Healing Traditions

Indigenous cultures worldwide have deep-rooted relationships with the plant kingdom. These cultures possess profound wisdom and intricate knowledge of local plants and their healing properties.

Native American healing traditions, for example, utilize plants for both physical and spiritual well-being. Herbal remedies are intricately tied to their cultural practices and are passed down through generations.

Similarly, African traditional medicine relies heavily on the use of herbs and plant-based remedies. Indigenous healers, known as traditional healers or herbalists, hold a wealth of knowledge about the medicinal properties of plants and their application in treating various conditions.

Indigenous Australian healing traditions, such as bush medicine, draw upon the abundant flora of the land. The Indigenous people of Australia have a deep understanding of the unique properties and uses of local plants for healing and spiritual purposes.

## 4.Herbals and Botanical Compendiums

Throughout history, herbal knowledge has been meticulously documented in herbals and botanical compendiums. These texts served as references for herbalists and physicians, providing detailed descriptions of plants and their medicinal properties.

One of the most influential herbal texts is "De Materia Medica" by Dioscorides, written in the 1st century AD. This comprehensive work cataloged over 600 plants and their therapeutic uses, serving as a foundational reference for herbal medicine.

During the Middle Ages and Renaissance, herbal compendiums continued to emerge. John Gerard's "Herball" and Nicholas Culpeper's "The English Physitian" became enduring classics, offering valuable insights into herbal medicine during their respective time periods. These texts not only described the medicinal properties of herbs but also provided instructions for their preparation and administration.

Botanical gardens also played a crucial role in the advancement of herbal knowledge. These gardens served as living repositories of medicinal plants, allowing herbalists and botanists to study, cultivate, and experiment with various species. The establishment of notable botanical gardens, such as the Botanical Garden of Padua in Italy and the Chelsea Physic Garden in England, contributed to the expansion of herbal knowledge and the development of botanical medicine.

## 5.The Renaissance and the Birth of Modern Medicine

The Renaissance marked a significant shift in the understanding and practice of medicine. It was during this period that a renewed interest in scientific inquiry and exploration emerged, leading to groundbreaking advancements in various fields, including herbal medicine.

Herbalists like John Gerard and Nicholas Culpeper played pivotal roles in disseminating herbal knowledge to the general public. Gerard's "Herball" became one of the most widely read herbals of the time, presenting detailed information on hundreds of plants and their uses.

Culpeper's "The English Physitian" challenged the prevailing medical establishment by making herbal medicine accessible to the common people. He believed that knowledge of herbal remedies should be shared with everyone, not just the privileged few. Culpeper's work not only provided information on medicinal plants but also included astrological correspondences and insights into the energetics of herbs.

## 6.Revival of Herbal Medicine

In the 19th and 20th centuries, as the influence of synthetic drugs grew, there was a resurgence of interest in herbal medicine. Many individuals sought alternatives to the side effects and limitations of conventional medicine, leading to a renewed appreciation for traditional healing practices.

Herbalists like Samuel Thomson in the United States and Maria Treben in Europe gained popularity for their herbal remedies and natural healing approaches. They advocated for the use of herbs in maintaining health and treating various ailments.

The late 20th century saw a vibrant resurgence of herbalism, often referred to as the modern herbal renaissance. Figures like Rosemary Gladstar and Susun Weed championed herbal medicine through their writings, teachings, and advocacy for self-care and holistic healing.

Today, herbal medicine continues to evolve and adapt. It integrates traditional wisdom with scientific research, emphasizing the importance of evidence-based practice and safety considerations. Herbalists, researchers, and healthcare providers work collaboratively to explore the potential of herbs in promoting well-being and supporting children's health.

## 1.2 Herbal Medicine Today: Benefits and Precautions

In today's modern world, herbal medicine continues to hold a vital place in healthcare practices, especially when it comes to children's health. Understanding the benefits and precautions of herbal medicine is essential for parents and caregivers seeking safe and effective natural remedies for their children.

1. Natural and Holistic Approach
   - Herbal medicine embraces a natural and holistic approach to health, considering the whole person rather than focusing solely on symptoms.
   - It recognizes the interconnectedness of the body, mind, and spirit, aiming to restore balance and promote overall well-being.

2. Gentle and Nurturing
   - Herbal remedies are often gentler on a child's delicate system

compared to potent pharmaceutical drugs.

- They can provide relief for common childhood ailments without causing harsh side effects or disruption to the body's natural processes.

3. Supporting the Body's Innate Healing Abilities

- Herbal medicine works with the body's innate healing abilities, stimulating and supporting its natural processes.
- It aims to address the root cause of an issue, rather than merely alleviating symptoms, promoting long-term healing and wellness.

4. Wide Range of Health Benefits

- Herbal remedies offer a wide range of health benefits for children, addressing various conditions such as respiratory issues, digestive discomfort, immune support, and emotional well-being.

- They can provide relief from common ailments like coughs, colds, digestive upsets, skin irritations, and anxiety.

5. Personalized Approach

- Herbal medicine allows for a personalized approach, taking into account each child's unique constitution, symptoms, and health history.

- It recognizes that what works for one child may not be suitable for another, emphasizing the importance of individualized care.

## Precautions and Safety Considerations

While herbal medicine can be highly beneficial for children, it is essential to approach its use with caution and respect for safety considerations.

1. Consultation with Healthcare Professionals
   - It is recommended to consult with a healthcare professional experienced in herbal medicine, such as a pediatrician or qualified

herbalist, before using herbs for children.

- They can provide guidance, ensure compatibility with existing treatments, and monitor for potential interactions or contraindications.

2. Age and Developmental Stage

- Children's bodies are still developing, and their physiological responses may differ from those of adults.
- Age-appropriate dosages and formulations should be used, and certain herbs may not be suitable for infants or young children.

3. Quality and Sourcing of Herbs

- It is important to source high-quality herbs from reputable suppliers to ensure their safety and efficacy.
- Organic and sustainably sourced herbs are preferred, as they reduce the risk of exposure to pesticides or contaminants.

4. Allergies and Sensitivities
   - Children may have allergies or sensitivities to specific herbs or plant families.
   - Care should be taken to identify any known allergies or sensitivities and avoid the use of herbs that may trigger an adverse reaction.

5. Adherence to Recommended Dosages

- Following recommended dosages is crucial to ensure the safe and effective use of herbal remedies.
- Dosages should be adjusted based on the child's age, weight, and individual response.

6. Monitoring for Adverse Reactions

- While rare, some children may experience adverse reactions to herbs.
- It is important to monitor for any unexpected symptoms or changes and discontinue use if adverse reactions occur.

By understanding the benefits and precautions of herbal medicine, parents and caregivers can make informed decisions and provide safe, effective, and nurturing care for their children. Herbal medicine, when used appropriately and with proper

## 1.3 Safety Considerations and Dosage Guidelines for Children

When using herbal remedies for children, it is crucial to prioritize their safety and well-being. By following proper safety considerations, parents and caregivers can ensure the responsible and effective use of herbal medicine.

1. Consultation with Healthcare Professionals
   - Before using herbal remedies, especially if your child has an existing medical condition or is taking other medications, it is advisable to consult with a healthcare professional.
   - A pediatrician, naturopathic doctor, or qualified herbalist can provide guidance tailored to your child's specific needs and ensure the safe integration of herbal remedies into their healthcare regimen.

2. Age Appropriateness
   - Consider your child's age when selecting herbal remedies. Some

herbs may not be suitable for infants or very young children.

- Consult age-specific references or seek advice from professionals to determine which herbs are safe and appropriate for your child's age group.

3. Allergies and Sensitivities

- Take into account any known allergies or sensitivities your child may have when choosing herbal remedies.
- Carefully review the ingredients of herbal products to avoid potential allergens or substances that may trigger an adverse reaction.

4. Quality and Sourcing

- Choose high-quality herbal products from reputable sources to ensure safety and efficacy.
- Look for organic or wildcrafted herbs, as they are less likely to be contaminated with pesticides or other harmful substances.

5. Start with Simple Remedies

- For younger children or those new to herbal remedies, start with simple, gentle herbs that have a long history of safe use.
- Gradually introduce more complex remedies or combinations as your child's system becomes accustomed to herbal interventions.

6. Adhere to Recommended Dosages

- Always follow the recommended dosages provided by the product manufacturer or healthcare professional.
- Dosages for children are typically lower than those for adults and are based on factors such as age, weight, and individual response.

## Dosage Guidelines for Herbal Remedies in Children

Proper dosage is crucial to ensure the safe and effective use of herbal remedies in children. Dosage guidelines may vary depending on the child's age, weight, and the specific herb being used. The following general guidelines can help provide a starting point for determining appropriate dosages:

1. Infants (up to 1 year):

    - Herbal remedies for infants should be used under the guidance of a healthcare professional.
    - Dosages are typically very low and may involve the use of diluted herbal extracts or teas.

2. Toddlers and Preschoolers (1-5 years):
    - Dosages for this age group are still relatively low and may involve the use of teas, syrups, or glycerites.

- Herbal remedies should be administered in small, divided doses throughout the day.

3. School-Aged Children (6-12 years):

    - Dosages can be slightly higher than for younger children, but it is still important to start with lower doses and monitor their response.
    - Tinctures, capsules, teas, or topical applications may be appropriate depending on the child's preference and the nature of the condition being treated.

4. Teenagers (13-18 years):

- Teenagers can generally tolerate higher dosages, approaching adult dosages.
- It is still important to consider individual factors and start with lower doses, gradually increasing as necessary.

Dosages should always be adjusted based on the child's response and any specific recommendations provided by a healthcare professional. Keep in mind that each child is unique, and their response to herbal remedies may vary. Regular monitoring and open communication with healthcare professionals will help ensure

# Chapter 2

# Creating a Herbal Medicine Cabinet

## *2.1 Essential Herbs for Children's Well-being*

When it comes to promoting children's well-being, certain herbs have gained recognition for their gentle yet effective properties. These essential herbs can support various aspects of children's health, from boosting immunity to soothing digestive discomfort. Understanding their benefits and safe usage can empower parents and caregivers to harness the healing power of herbs for their children.

1.  Chamomile (Matricaria chamomilla):
    - Chamomile is renowned for its calming and soothing properties, making it a popular herb for promoting relaxation and restful sleep in children.
    - It can also be used to alleviate digestive discomfort, such as colic or upset stomach.

2.  Echinacea (Echinacea purpurea):
    - Echinacea is a powerful immune-supporting herb that can help strengthen a child's natural defenses against common infections, such as colds and flu.

- It is often used preventively during the cold and flu season or at the first sign of illness.

3. Elderberry (Sambucus nigra):
    - Elderberry is well-known for its immune-enhancing properties and is commonly used to support the body's defense against viral infections, particularly during the cold and flu season.
    - It can be taken in syrup or gummy form, making it easier for children to consume.

4. Ginger (Zingiber officinale):
    - Ginger is a warming herb with anti-inflammatory and digestive benefits.

- It can help relieve nausea, motion sickness, and digestive discomfort, making it particularly useful for children experiencing tummy troubles.

5. Lemon Balm (Melissa officinalis):
- Lemon balm is a gentle herb known for its calming and mood-supporting properties.
- It can be used to ease anxiety, promote relaxation, and support a positive mood in children.

6. Marshmallow Root (Althaea officinalis):
- Marshmallow root is a demulcent herb that can help soothe irritated mucous membranes, making it useful for

relieving coughs and throat irritation in children.

- It can be consumed in the form of herbal teas or syrups.

7. Peppermint (Mentha piperita):
- Peppermint is a refreshing herb with digestive benefits.
- It can help alleviate digestive discomfort, including bloating, gas, and stomachaches, making it suitable for children with digestive issues.

8. Calendula (Calendula officinalis):
    - Calendula is a gentle and soothing herb often used in topical preparations for skin irritations and minor wounds.

- It can be applied as a cream, ointment, or infused oil to soothe and promote the healing of minor cuts, scrapes, rashes, and insect bites.

9. Valerian (Valeriana officinalis):

- Valerian is a calming herb that can be used to promote relaxation and improve sleep quality in children with occasional sleep disturbances.
- It is commonly used as a bedtime herb in small, appropriate doses.

10. Catnip (Nepeta cataria):

- Catnip is a gentle herb known for its calming effects on the nervous system.

- It can help promote relaxation, reduce restlessness, and soothe an upset stomach in children.

Remember, when using herbal remedies for children, it is essential to consider the child's age, weight, individual response, and any specific health conditions. Always consult with a healthcare professional or qualified herbalist for guidance on the appropriate use and dosages of herbs for your child's specific needs.

Exploring the use of these essential herbs can provide parents and caregivers with natural tools to support their children's well-being and nurture their health in a gentle and holistic manner.

## 2.2 Sourcing and Growing Medicinal Herbs

When using medicinal herbs for children's health, it is crucial to source high-quality herbs from reputable suppliers. Here are some considerations for sourcing medicinal herbs:

1. Reputable Suppliers:

- Look for suppliers who prioritize quality, sustainability, and ethical practices in their herb sourcing.
- Research the reputation and certifications of the supplier to ensure they meet industry standards.

2. Organic and Sustainable:

- Choose organic herbs whenever possible to minimize exposure to pesticides, herbicides, and other potentially harmful substances.
- Opt for sustainably sourced herbs to support environmental conservation and ensure long-term availability.

3. Quality Testing:

- Inquire about the quality testing practices of the supplier, such as testing for purity, potency, and absence of contaminants.

- Certifications like Good Manufacturing Practices (GMP) ensure adherence to quality standards.

4. Local and Seasonal:

- Consider sourcing herbs locally and seasonally, as this promotes freshness and supports local farmers and herbalists.
- Local herbs may also be more suited to the regional needs and climate.

5. Trusted Herbal Companies:

- Look for well-established herbal companies with a history of reliable products and positive customer feedback.

- Read reviews and testimonials from other customers to gain insights into the quality and efficacy of their products.

## Growing Medicinal Herbs

Growing medicinal herbs at home can be a rewarding and sustainable way to ensure a fresh and readily available supply. Here are some tips for growing medicinal herbs:

1. Selecting the Right Herbs:

- Choose medicinal herbs that are well-suited to your climate, available space, and growing conditions.

- Consider the specific health needs of your children and prioritize herbs that will be most beneficial to their well-being.

2. Sunlight and Soil Requirements:

- Most medicinal herbs thrive in full sunlight, so select a sunny location for your herb garden or consider container gardening.
- Ensure the soil is well-drained, rich in organic matter, and suitable for the specific herbs you are growing.

3. Seed or Seedling Selection:

- Decide whether to start your herbs from seeds or purchase seedlings.
- Starting from seeds allows for a wider variety of herbs, while seedlings provide a head start in the growing process.

4. Care and Maintenance:

- Regularly water and fertilize your herbs according to their specific needs.
- Monitor for pests and diseases and take appropriate measures to protect your plants.

5. Harvesting and Drying:

- Harvest herbs at the appropriate time, usually when the plant is in full bloom or when the desired plant parts are at their peak.
- Follow proper drying techniques to preserve the medicinal properties of the herbs.

6. Storage and Labeling:

- Store dried herbs in airtight containers, away from light and moisture.
- Label each container with the herb's name, date of harvest, and any other relevant information.

Growing your own medicinal herbs can be a fulfilling and sustainable way to ensure a readily available supply of high-quality herbs for your child's health needs. However, if you decide to grow your own herbs, it is still important to consult with a healthcare professional or qualified herbalist for guidance on their safe and appropriate use, especially for children.

By sourcing and growing medicinal herbs responsibly, you can have confidence in the quality, sustainability, and effectiveness of the herbs you use for supporting your children's health and well-being.

## 2.3 Herbal Preparation Techniques: Infusions, Tinctures, and More

Preparing herbal remedies involves various techniques to extract the beneficial compounds from medicinal herbs. Here are some common herbal preparation methods:

1. Herbal Infusions:

   - Infusions are made by steeping herbs in hot water to extract their medicinal properties.
   - Suitable for delicate parts of the plant, such as leaves and flowers.
   - Examples include herbal teas and floral waters.

## 2. Decoctions:

- Decoctions involve simmering tougher plant parts, such as roots, bark, or seeds, in water for an extended period.
- This method is used to extract the medicinal properties from tougher plant materials.
- Decoctions are often used for herbs with stronger active constituents.

## 3. Herbal Tinctures:

- Tinctures are concentrated liquid extracts of herbs, typically made using alcohol or a combination of alcohol and water.

- Tinctures have a longer shelf life and can be easily measured for precise dosing.
- They are a popular and convenient form of herbal medicine.

4. Herbal Syrups:

- Syrups are made by combining herbal infusions or decoctions with sweeteners, such as honey or maple syrup.
- Syrups are a pleasant and palatable way to administer herbal remedies, especially for children.

- They are often used for respiratory conditions, coughs, and immune support.

5. Herbal Oils:

- Herbal oils are made by infusing herbs in carrier oils, such as olive oil or coconut oil.
- They are used topically for various purposes, such as soothing skin irritations or as a base for herbal salves and creams.

6. Herbal Salves and Balms:

- Salves and balms are semi-solid preparations made by combining herbal oils with beeswax or other solidifying agents.

- They are applied topically to nourish the skin, promote healing, or provide relief for minor cuts, burns, or insect bites.

7. Herbal Poultices and Compresses:

- Poultices involve applying a moist herbal preparation directly to the skin.
- Compresses are made by soaking a cloth or compress in an herbal infusion or decoction and applying it to the affected area.
- These external applications can provide localized relief for

muscle aches, bruises, or skin conditions.

8. Herbal Capsules and Tablets:

- Herbal powders or extracts can be encapsulated or compressed into tablets for convenient oral administration.
- Capsules and tablets are commonly used for herbs with a strong taste or for those who prefer a more standardized dosage form.

Remember to follow specific recipes, guidelines, and dosage recommendations when preparing herbal remedies using these techniques. It is also essential to store prepared herbal preparations properly to maintain their potency and effectiveness.

## 2.4 Tools and Supplies for Herbal Remedies

When engaging in herbal remedies for children's health, having the right tools and supplies is essential for effective preparation and administration. Here are some essential tools and supplies for herbal remedies:

1. Mortar and Pestle:

   - A mortar and pestle are used for grinding and crushing herbs, seeds, and other plant materials to create herbal powders or for extracting the active constituents.

- Choose a sturdy and appropriately sized mortar and pestle for your needs.

2. Herb Grinder or Coffee Grinder:

- An herb grinder or coffee grinder can be used as an alternative to a mortar and pestle for grinding herbs into finer powders.
- Ensure it is specifically dedicated to herb grinding to avoid cross-contamination of flavors.

3. Kitchen Scale:

- A kitchen scale helps accurately measure the weight of herbs and other ingredients when following herbal recipes.

- It is particularly useful for preparing tinctures, where precise measurements are crucial.

4. Measuring Spoons and Cups:

- Have a set of measuring spoons and cups specifically designated for herbal remedies to ensure accurate dosing of herbs, oils, and other ingredients.

5. Strainers and Cheesecloth:

- Strainers and cheesecloth are used to filter herbal infusions, decoctions, or tinctures, separating the liquid from the plant material.
- Opt for fine-mesh strainers and high-quality cheesecloth to ensure efficient filtration.

6. Glass Jars and Bottles:

- Glass jars and bottles are ideal for storing dried herbs, herbal preparations, tinctures, oils, and syrups.
- Choose dark-colored glass containers to protect the contents from light degradation.

7. Labels and Markers:

- Labels and markers are essential for accurately identifying and labeling your herbal preparations.
- Clearly label each container with the herb's name, preparation date, and any specific dosage or usage instructions.

## Additional Supplies for Herbal Remedies

1. Organic Herbs:

- Source high-quality, organic herbs from reputable suppliers or grow your own medicinal herbs.
- Choose herbs that are suitable for your child's specific health needs.

2. Alcohol and Carrier Oils:

- Alcohol, such as vodka or brandy, is commonly used for making tinctures.
- Carrier oils, such as olive oil or coconut oil, are used for herbal infusions, oils, salves, and balms.
- Ensure the alcohol and oils are of good quality and appropriate for herbal preparations.

3. Sweeteners:

- Natural sweeteners like honey or maple syrup are often used in herbal syrups to improve taste and palatability for children.

4. Clean Water:

- Use clean, filtered water for preparing herbal infusions, decoctions, and other herbal remedies.
- Water quality can affect the final outcome and safety of your preparations.

5. Storage Containers:

- Have a variety of airtight glass containers, jars, and bottles for storing dried herbs, herbal preparations, and infused oils.
- Choose sizes that accommodate your specific needs.

6. Reference Books and Resources:

- Invest in reliable herbal reference books or access reputable online resources for accurate information on herbs, dosage guidelines, and preparation techniques.
- Stay informed about potential interactions, contraindications, and safety considerations.

Having the necessary tools and supplies for herbal remedies will help you create and administer herbal preparations confidently and effectively. Remember to keep your tools and supplies clean and organized to maintain the quality and safety of your herbal remedies.

# Chapter 3

# <u>Boosting Immunity and</u> <u>Warding off Illness</u>

## *3.1 Immune-Boosting Herbs and Remedies*

A strong immune system is vital for children's overall well-being and their ability to fight off infections. Here are some immune-boosting herbs and remedies that can support your child's immune health:

1. Elderberry (Sambucus nigra):

- Elderberry is well-known for its immune-enhancing properties and is rich in antioxidants and vitamins.
- Elderberry syrup or gummies can be taken preventively during the cold and flu season or at the first sign of illness.

2. Echinacea (Echinacea purpurea):

- Echinacea is a powerful herb that can help strengthen the immune system and support the body's natural defense mechanisms.
- It is commonly used to prevent and reduce the duration of colds and respiratory infections.

3. Astragalus (Astragalus membranaceus):

- Astragalus is an adaptogenic herb that helps support and balance the immune system.
- It is often used as a tonic to promote overall immune health and resilience.

4. Garlic (Allium sativum):

- Garlic is a potent immune booster with antimicrobial and antiviral properties.
- Including garlic in your child's diet or using garlic supplements can help enhance their immune response.

5. Reishi Mushroom (Ganoderma lucidum):

- Reishi mushroom is a medicinal mushroom known for its immune-modulating effects.
- It can be consumed as a tea, tincture, or in powdered form to support immune function.

6. Calendula (Calendula officinalis):

- Calendula is an immune-supportive herb that also has antimicrobial and anti-inflammatory properties.

- It can be used in teas, tinctures, or as a topical cream for minor skin irritations or infections.

7. Ginger (Zingiber officinale):

- Ginger is a warming herb with immune-boosting properties and anti-inflammatory benefits.
- It can be consumed as a tea or added to foods and beverages to support immune function.

8. Lemon Balm (Melissa officinalis):

- Lemon balm is a calming herb that also possesses antiviral properties.

- It can be used in teas or herbal preparations to support the immune system and reduce stress.

9. Probiotics:

- Probiotics are beneficial bacteria that support a healthy immune system by promoting a balanced gut microbiome.
- Probiotic supplements or fermented foods like yogurt and kefir can be included in your child's diet.

10. Vitamin C:

- While not an herb, vitamin C is essential for immune health and can be found in citrus fruits, berries, and leafy greens.
- Ensure your child's diet includes ample sources of vitamin C or consider supplementation if needed.

11.  Licorice Root (Glycyrrhiza glabra):

- Licorice root is an immune-supportive herb with anti-inflammatory and antiviral properties.
- It can be used to support the respiratory system and soothe coughs.

## Immune-Boosting Herbal Remedies

1. Immune-Boosting Herbal Tea:

- Create a blend using a combination of immune-boosting herbs such as astragalus, echinacea, and ginger.
- Steep the herbs in hot water and sweeten with honey for a soothing and immune-enhancing tea.

2. Elderberry Syrup:

- Prepare a homemade elderberry syrup using dried or fresh elderberries, honey, and immune-enhancing herbs.

- Elderberry syrup can be taken daily during cold and flu season to support the immune system.

3. Immune-Enhancing Tincture:

   - Create an immune-enhancing tincture by combining immune-boosting herbs like echinacea, astragalus, and reishi mushroom.
   - Use a blend of alcohol and water to extract the medicinal properties and take as directed.

4. Garlic and Honey Infusion:

- Crush fresh garlic cloves and mix with honey to create an immune-boosting infusion.
- Allow the mixture to infuse for several hours before consuming a small amount daily.

5. Immune-Supporting Herbal Soup:

- Prepare a nourishing soup using immune-boosting herbs and ingredients such as garlic, astragalus, and medicinal mushrooms.
- Simmer the herbs and other ingredients in a flavorful broth for a comforting and immune-supporting meal.

6. Respiratory Support Herbal Steam:

- Create a herbal steam inhalation to support respiratory health and boost the immune system.
- Add immune-enhancing herbs such as eucalyptus, thyme, and rosemary to a bowl of hot water, cover your child's head with a towel, and have them inhale the steam for a few minutes.

7. Immune-Boosting Herbal Bath:

- Infuse a warm bath with immune-boosting herbs like calendula, chamomile, and lavender.

- Allow your child to soak in the herbal bath to promote relaxation, relieve congestion, and support overall immune function.

8. Immune-Supporting Herbal Gummies:

- Create homemade herbal gummies using immune-boosting herbs like elderberry and echinacea.
- Combine herbal infusions or powders with gelatin and natural sweeteners to make delicious and immune-enhancing gummy treats.

It is important to note that individual responses to herbs may vary, and it is always advisable to consult with a healthcare professional or qualified herbalist before starting any herbal regimen, especially for children with specific health conditions or those taking medications.

## 3.2 Herbal Support for Common Childhood Illnesses

Children often experience common illnesses such as colds, coughs, fevers, digestive issues, and skin irritations. Here are some herbal remedies that can provide support and relief for these common childhood ailments:

1. Colds and Congestion:

- Eucalyptus (Eucalyptus globulus) and Peppermint (Mentha piperita) are herbs with decongestant properties.
- Use them in steam inhalations or as essential oils diluted in carrier oils for chest rubs.

2. Coughs:

- Marshmallow (Althaea officinalis) and Thyme (Thymus vulgaris) are soothing herbs that can help alleviate coughs.
- Make herbal infusions or syrups using these herbs and give them in appropriate doses.

3. Fevers:

- Elderflower (Sambucus nigra) and Yarrow (Achillea millefolium) are herbs known for their diaphoretic properties, helping to promote sweating and reduce fevers.
- Prepare herbal infusions or use them in bath blends to support the body's natural response to fever.

4. Digestive Issues:

- Chamomile (Matricaria chamomilla) and Ginger (Zingiber officinale) are soothing herbs that can help with digestive discomfort, including indigestion and stomachaches.

- Prepare herbal teas or give ginger in small, grated amounts for relief.

5. Diarrhea:

- Blackberry (Rubus fruticosus) and Raspberry (Rubus idaeus) leaves have astringent properties that can help reduce diarrhea.
- Prepare herbal infusions and offer small, frequent sips to rehydrate and soothe the digestive system.

6. Skin Irritations:

- Calendula (Calendula officinalis) and Lavender (Lavandula angustifolia) are gentle and soothing herbs for skin irritations, including rashes, insect bites, and minor cuts.
- Apply infused oils, creams, or herbal compresses to the affected area for relief.

7. Earaches:

- Mullein (Verbascum thapsus) and Garlic (Allium sativum) have antibacterial and anti-inflammatory properties that may help alleviate earaches.
- Consult a healthcare professional before using any herbal remedies

for earaches, especially if the eardrum is perforated or if there are severe symptoms.

Always ensure proper dosing and follow age-appropriate guidelines when using herbal remedies for children. If your child's symptoms persist or worsen, seek medical advice or consult with a qualified healthcare professional or herbalist.

Additionally, it is important to note that herbal remedies should not replace medical treatment for serious illnesses or emergencies. Use herbs as a supportive measure in conjunction with appropriate medical care.

## 3.3 Preventive Measures: Herbs for a Healthy Immune System

Maintaining a healthy immune system is essential for preventing illnesses and promoting overall well-being in children. Here are some herbs that can support a robust immune system:

1. Ginseng (Panax ginseng):

   - Ginseng is an adaptogenic herb known for its immune-modulating properties.
   - It can enhance the body's natural defenses and support overall immune health.

2. Holy Basil (Ocimum sanctum):

- Holy Basil, also known as Tulsi, is an herb revered for its immune-stimulating and stress-relieving properties.
- It can help strengthen the immune system and promote a balanced response to stress.

3. Ashwagandha (Withania somnifera):

- Ashwagandha is an adaptogenic herb that supports the body's ability to adapt to stressors, thereby promoting overall immune health.

- It can help enhance the immune response and reduce the risk of infections.

4. Licorice Root (Glycyrrhiza glabra):

- Licorice root has immune-enhancing properties and can support respiratory health.
- It can be used in teas or herbal preparations to promote a healthy immune system.

5. Cat's Claw (Uncaria tomentosa):

- Cat's Claw is an immune-stimulating herb that can

help enhance the body's natural defense mechanisms.

- It is commonly used to support the immune system and protect against infections.

6. Astragalus (Astragalus membranaceus):

- Astragalus is an adaptogenic herb that supports immune health and promotes resilience.
- It can help strengthen the immune system and protect against respiratory infections.

7. Oregano (Origanum vulgare):

- Oregano is a potent herb with antimicrobial and immune-stimulating properties.
- It can be used as a culinary herb or taken as a supplement to support immune function.

8. Elderberry (Sambucus nigra):

- Elderberry is well-known for its immune-boosting properties due to its high antioxidant content.
- It can be consumed as a syrup or in other forms to strengthen the immune system.

9. Garlic (Allium sativum):

- Garlic is a potent immune booster with antimicrobial and antiviral properties.
- Including garlic in your child's diet can help support their immune response.

10. Green Tea (Camellia sinensis):

- Green tea is rich in antioxidants and polyphenols that can support immune health.
- Encourage your child to drink green tea or use it in herbal preparations for immune support.

Incorporating these immune-supporting herbs into your child's diet and wellness routine, along with a balanced diet, regular exercise, adequate sleep, and good hygiene practices, can help strengthen their immune system and reduce the risk of illness.

Remember to consult with a healthcare professional or qualified herbalist before introducing herbs to your child's routine, especially if they have underlying health conditions or are taking medications.

By incorporating these preventive measures and herbs into your child's lifestyle, you can help support their immune system and promote their overall health and well-being.

# Chapter 4

## Soothing Digestive Discomforts

### *4.1 Gentle Herbs for Digestive Health*

Maintaining a healthy digestive system is crucial for children's overall well-being. Here are some gentle herbs that can support digestive health in children:

1. Chamomile (Matricaria chamomilla):

    - Chamomile is a calming herb that can help soothe digestive discomfort, including indigestion, bloating, and stomachaches.

- Prepare chamomile tea or use it in herbal blends designed for digestive support.

2. Peppermint (Mentha piperita):

- Peppermint is a cooling herb with carminative properties, making it useful for relieving digestive issues such as gas, bloating, and indigestion.
- Offer peppermint tea or diluted peppermint oil in appropriate doses to alleviate discomfort.

3. Fennel (Foeniculum vulgare):

- Fennel is a digestive herb commonly used to relieve colic, gas, and stomach cramps in children.
- Infuse fennel seeds in hot water to make a gentle tea or use it in herbal preparations for digestive relief.

4. Ginger (Zingiber officinale):

- Ginger is a warming herb that can aid digestion, reduce nausea, and relieve stomach discomfort.
- Offer ginger tea, grated ginger in foods or beverages, or ginger candies for digestive support.

5. Slippery Elm (Ulmus rubra):

- Slippery Elm is a demulcent herb that forms a soothing gel when mixed with water, providing relief for irritated digestive linings.

- Use powdered slippery elm to make a porridge-like mixture or as an ingredient in herbal remedies for digestive support.

6. Lemon Balm (Melissa officinalis):

- Lemon Balm is a gentle herb with calming properties that can help soothe digestive upset, especially due to nervousness or stress.

- Prepare lemon balm tea or incorporate it into herbal blends for digestive support.

7. Dandelion (Taraxacum officinale):

- Dandelion is a bitter herb that stimulates digestion, supports liver function, and aids in detoxification.
- Offer dandelion tea or incorporate dandelion leaves in salads or other culinary preparations.

8. Licorice Root (Glycyrrhiza glabra):

- Licorice root is an herb known for its soothing and

anti-inflammatory properties, making it useful for relieving digestive discomfort and promoting a healthy digestive system.

- Use licorice root in herbal preparations or offer licorice tea in appropriate doses.

Remember to consider your child's specific needs and consult with a healthcare professional or qualified herbalist before introducing new herbs or herbal preparations, especially if your child has underlying health conditions or is taking medications.

In addition to incorporating these gentle herbs, encourage your child to have a balanced and fiber-rich diet, stay hydrated, engage in regular physical activity, and practice mindful eating habits for optimal digestive health.

## 4.2 Herbal Remedies for Upset Stomachs and Colic

Upset stomachs and colic can cause significant discomfort in children. Here are some herbal remedies that can help soothe these conditions:

1. Chamomile (Matricaria chamomilla):

    - Chamomile is a gentle herb known for its calming and anti-inflammatory properties.

- Prepare chamomile tea and offer it to your child in small sips to help soothe an upset stomach and reduce colic symptoms.

2. Fennel (Foeniculum vulgare):

- Fennel is a carminative herb that can aid digestion, reduce gas, and relieve colic symptoms.
- Infuse fennel seeds in hot water to make a soothing tea or use fennel water to ease stomach discomfort.

3. Peppermint (Mentha piperita):

- Peppermint is a cooling herb with antispasmodic properties that can help alleviate stomach cramps and colic.

- Offer diluted peppermint tea to your child or apply diluted peppermint oil in a clockwise massage motion on their abdomen.

4. Lemon Balm (Melissa officinalis):

- Lemon Balm is a gentle herb known for its calming properties and ability to relieve digestive upset.
- Prepare lemon balm tea and offer it to your child to soothe an upset stomach and reduce colic symptoms.

5. Ginger (Zingiber officinale):

- Ginger is a warming herb with anti-inflammatory properties that can ease stomach discomfort and colic.
- Offer ginger tea or diluted ginger oil in appropriate doses to your child to help relieve symptoms.

6. Catnip (Nepeta cataria):

- Catnip is a calming herb that can help soothe an upset stomach and reduce colic symptoms.
- Prepare catnip tea and offer it to your child to promote relaxation and ease digestive discomfort.

7. Marshmallow Root (Althaea officinalis):

- Marshmallow root is a demulcent herb that can help soothe and protect the digestive lining, reducing stomach irritation.
- Prepare marshmallow root tea or use it as an ingredient in herbal blends for digestive support.

Remember to consult with a healthcare professional or qualified herbalist before using herbal remedies, especially for young infants or children with specific health conditions or sensitivities.

In addition to using these herbal remedies, it's important to address other potential causes of upset stomachs and colic, such as food intolerances, allergies, or excessive air swallowing during feeding. Observe your child's symptoms, keep a food diary, and seek medical advice if symptoms persist or worsen.

## 4.3 *Supporting Healthy Digestion in Children*

Maintaining healthy digestion is vital for children's overall well-being and nutrient absorption. Here are some strategies and herbal remedies to support healthy digestion in children:

1. Balanced and Fiber-Rich Diet:

- Encourage your child to consume a diet rich in fruits, vegetables, whole grains, and fiber.
- Fiber promotes regular bowel movements and helps prevent constipation.

2. Hydration:

- Ensure your child stays adequately hydrated by drinking plenty of water throughout the day.
- Sufficient hydration supports optimal digestion and prevents constipation.

3. Mindful Eating Habits:

- Encourage your child to eat slowly, chew their food thoroughly, and pay attention to their body's cues of hunger and fullness.
- Mindful eating promotes proper digestion and prevents overeating.

4. Probiotics:

- Probiotics are beneficial bacteria that support a healthy gut microbiome.
- Consider incorporating probiotic-rich foods like yogurt or fermented foods into your child's diet or consult with a healthcare professional about

probiotic supplements suitable for children.

5. Herbal Digestive Tonics:

- Gentle herbal tonics can aid digestion and support overall digestive health.
- Herbs like Dandelion root, Burdock root, and Yellow Dock root can be used in herbal blends or as tea to promote healthy digestion.

6. Peppermint (Mentha piperita):

- Peppermint is a digestive herb that can help alleviate digestive discomfort, including gas, bloating, and indigestion.

- Offer peppermint tea or diluted peppermint oil in appropriate doses to your child to aid digestion.

7. Ginger (Zingiber officinale):

- Ginger is a warming herb that can support healthy digestion, relieve nausea, and soothe an upset stomach.
- Incorporate ginger in meals, offer ginger tea, or use ginger candies to promote optimal digestion.

8. Papaya (Carica papaya):

- Papaya contains an enzyme called papain that aids in digestion by breaking down proteins.
- Offer fresh papaya as a snack or include it in smoothies to support healthy digestion.

9. Aloe Vera (Aloe barbadensis):

- Aloe Vera has soothing properties that can support the digestive system and promote regular bowel movements.
- Consult with a healthcare professional for appropriate aloe vera products suitable for children.

Remember to introduce herbs gradually, consider your child's individual sensitivities, and consult with a healthcare professional or qualified herbalist before introducing new herbs or herbal preparations.

In addition to these strategies, ensure your child engages in regular physical activity, gets enough sleep, and manages stress, as these factors also contribute to healthy digestion.

By implementing these practices and incorporating herbal remedies into your child's routine, you can support their healthy digestion, optimize nutrient absorption, and promote their overall digestive wellness.

# Chapter 5.

# <u>Nurturing Respiratory Health</u>

## *5.1 Herbal Allies for Respiratory Wellness*

Maintaining healthy respiratory function is crucial for children's well-being, especially during seasons when respiratory illnesses are more common. Here are some herbal allies that can support respiratory wellness in children:

1. Echinacea (Echinacea purpurea):

- Echinacea is an immune-stimulating herb that can help support respiratory health.
- It can be used preventively or at the onset of respiratory symptoms to boost the immune system.

2. Thyme (Thymus vulgaris):

- Thyme is an herb with antimicrobial and expectorant properties, making it beneficial for respiratory health.
- Prepare thyme tea or use it in steam inhalations to help soothe coughs and support healthy airways.

3. Mullein (Verbascum thapsus):

- Mullein is a respiratory tonic herb that can help soothe coughs, alleviate congestion, and promote respiratory wellness.
- Prepare mullein tea or use it in herbal blends designed for respiratory support.

4. Licorice Root (Glycyrrhiza glabra):

- Licorice root has expectorant and anti-inflammatory properties, making it helpful for respiratory conditions.
- Offer licorice tea or use it in herbal preparations to help soothe

coughs and support respiratory health.

5. Marshmallow Root (Althaea officinalis):

- Marshmallow root is a demulcent herb that can help soothe irritation in the respiratory system.
- Use marshmallow root in teas or herbal blends to provide gentle support for the respiratory system.

6. Plantain (Plantago spp.):

- Plantain is an herb known for its soothing and expectorant properties, making it beneficial for respiratory wellness.

- Use plantain leaf in teas or as an ingredient in herbal preparations to help relieve respiratory congestion and irritation.

7. Elderflower (Sambucus nigra):

- Elderflower has antimicrobial and anti-inflammatory properties that can support respiratory health.
- Prepare elderflower tea or use it in herbal blends to help alleviate respiratory congestion and discomfort.

8. Osha Root (Ligusticum porteri):

- Osha root is a respiratory herb traditionally used to support respiratory wellness.
- It can be used as a tincture or in herbal blends for respiratory support.

Remember to consult with a healthcare professional or qualified herbalist before using herbs, especially for children with specific respiratory conditions or allergies.

In addition to using herbal allies, encourage your child to practice good respiratory hygiene, such as covering their mouth and nose when coughing or sneezing, washing their hands regularly, and avoiding exposure to environmental pollutants.

## 5.2 Managing Coughs, Colds, and Congestion with Herbs

Coughs, colds, and congestion are common respiratory symptoms that can cause discomfort in children. Here are some herbal remedies to help manage these symptoms:

1. Eucalyptus (Eucalyptus globulus):

   - Eucalyptus is a powerful decongestant and expectorant that can help relieve respiratory congestion and coughs.
   - Use eucalyptus essential oil in a diffuser or add a few drops to a

bowl of hot water for steam inhalation.

2. Peppermint (Mentha piperita):

- Peppermint has soothing properties and can help alleviate coughs and clear congestion.
- Offer peppermint tea or diluted peppermint oil in appropriate doses to provide relief.

3. Lemon (Citrus limon):

- Lemon is rich in vitamin C and has antimicrobial properties, making it beneficial for colds and coughs.

- Squeeze fresh lemon juice into warm water and add a teaspoon of honey for a soothing drink.

4. Ginger (Zingiber officinale):

- Ginger is a warming herb with expectorant properties that can help relieve coughs and ease congestion.
- Offer ginger tea or incorporate ginger in meals to provide relief.

5. Honey:

- Honey has natural soothing properties and can help relieve coughs and sore throats.

- Offer a teaspoon of raw, organic honey to children above the age of one year.

6. Marshmallow Root (Althaea officinalis):

  - Marshmallow root is a demulcent herb that can help soothe irritated throats and alleviate coughs.
  - Use marshmallow root in teas or as an ingredient in herbal preparations for respiratory relief.

7. Calendula (Calendula officinalis):

  - Calendula has antimicrobial and anti-inflammatory properties that can support respiratory health.

- Use calendula in herbal blends or as a gargle to soothe sore throats.

8. Slippery Elm (Ulmus rubra):

   - Slippery Elm is a demulcent herb that can help relieve coughs and soothe irritated airways.
   - Use slippery elm lozenges or incorporate powdered slippery elm into herbal preparations.

Remember to consider your child's age, any underlying health conditions, and consult with a healthcare professional or qualified herbalist before using herbal remedies.

In addition to herbal support, encourage your child to rest, drink plenty of fluids, and maintain a healthy diet to support their immune system and aid in recovery.

## 5.3 *Promoting Healthy Breathing in Children*

Healthy breathing is essential for optimal physical and mental well-being in children. Here are some strategies and herbal remedies to promote healthy breathing:

1. Indoor Air Quality:

  - Ensure that the indoor environment where your child spends most of their time has good air quality.

- Keep the area well-ventilated, free from smoke or strong odors, and consider using air purifiers or plants that improve air quality.

2. Allergy Management:

- Identify and address any potential allergens that may trigger respiratory symptoms in your child, such as dust mites, pet dander, or pollen.
- Maintain a clean and allergen-free environment, use dust mite covers on mattresses and pillows, and consider air filters if needed.

3. Regular Physical Activity:

- Encourage your child to engage in regular physical activity to promote lung health and strengthen their respiratory muscles.
- Activities like running, swimming, and cycling can help improve lung capacity and overall breathing efficiency.

4. Breathing Exercises:

- Teach your child simple breathing exercises to enhance lung capacity and promote deep, relaxed breathing.
- Deep belly breathing, pursed lip breathing, and alternate nostril

breathing are some techniques that can be beneficial.

5. Aromatherapy:

- Certain essential oils can help promote healthy breathing and clear respiratory passages.
- Eucalyptus, peppermint, lavender, and tea tree oil are commonly used for their respiratory benefits. Dilute them appropriately and use them in diffusers or steam inhalations.

6. Herbal Respiratory Tonics:

- Herbal blends specifically formulated to support respiratory health can be beneficial for children.

- Look for blends containing herbs like elecampane, hyssop, horehound, and lobelia, which have traditionally been used to enhance lung function and promote healthy breathing.

7. Breathing Exercises through Play:

- Incorporate breathing exercises into fun activities and games to make it enjoyable for your child.
- For example, blowing bubbles or using a pinwheel can encourage deep breathing and lung expansion.

8. Encourage Fresh Air:

- Spend time outdoors in nature to allow your child to breathe in fresh air.
- Outdoor activities provide an opportunity for deeper breathing and exposure to natural elements that can support respiratory wellness.

Remember to tailor these strategies to your child's age and individual needs. Consult with a healthcare professional or qualified herbalist for guidance, especially if your child has respiratory conditions or allergies.

By implementing these strategies and incorporating herbal remedies, you can promote healthy breathing in your child, supporting their respiratory wellness and overall vitality.

# Chapter 6

# <u>Calming the Mind and</u> <u>Promoting Restful Sleep</u>

## *6.1 Herbal Solutions for Anxiety and Stress*

Anxiety and stress can affect children's emotional well-being and overall quality of life. Here are some herbal solutions to help manage anxiety and stress in children:

1. Chamomile (Matricaria chamomilla):

- Chamomile is a calming herb that can help soothe anxiety and promote relaxation.
- Offer chamomile tea or incorporate chamomile in herbal blends designed to alleviate anxiety.

2. Lemon Balm (Melissa officinalis):

- Lemon balm has gentle sedative properties and can help reduce anxiety and promote a sense of calm.
- Offer lemon balm tea or use it as an ingredient in herbal preparations to support emotional well-being.

3. Lavender (Lavandula angustifolia):

- Lavender is renowned for its calming and soothing properties.
- Use lavender essential oil in a diffuser, offer lavender-infused bath products, or create sachets with dried lavender for a calming aroma.

4. Passionflower (Passiflora incarnata):

- Passionflower is a relaxing herb that can help reduce anxiety and promote a sense of tranquility.
- Offer passionflower tea or use it as an ingredient in herbal preparations designed for stress relief.

5. Valerian (Valeriana officinalis):

- Valerian is a sedative herb that can help calm anxiety and improve sleep quality.
- Use valerian root in teas or consider valerian supplements under the guidance of a healthcare professional.

6. Adaptogenic Herbs:

- Adaptogens like Ashwagandha (Withania somnifera) and Rhodiola (Rhodiola rosea) can help the body adapt to stress and support emotional well-being.

- Consult with a healthcare professional or qualified herbalist for appropriate dosages and preparations.

7. Mindfulness Teas:

- Create herbal tea blends using calming herbs like chamomile, lemon balm, and lavender.
- Encourage your child to sit quietly, savor the tea, and practice mindfulness to promote relaxation.

8. Herbal Baths:

- Create a calming bath experience by adding dried herbs like chamomile, lavender, and lemon balm to warm bathwater.

- The soothing aroma and herbal properties can help alleviate stress and promote relaxation.

Remember that managing anxiety and stress in children may require a holistic approach that includes open communication, emotional support, and appropriate professional guidance if needed.

## 6.2 Bedtime Rituals: Herbs for Peaceful Sleep

Establishing a soothing bedtime routine is crucial for promoting peaceful sleep in children. Incorporating herbs known for their calming properties can enhance the relaxation process. Here are some herbs to consider for a peaceful sleep ritual:

1. Lavender (Lavandula angustifolia):

   - Lavender is a well-known herb with relaxing properties that can help induce a sense of calm before sleep.
   - Use lavender essential oil in a diffuser or add a few drops to a bedtime bath for a soothing aroma.

2. Chamomile (Matricaria chamomilla):

- Chamomile is a gentle herb that can promote relaxation and support restful sleep.
- Offer chamomile tea or incorporate chamomile in a bedtime blend to help your child unwind.

3. Lemon Balm (Melissa officinalis):

- Lemon balm has calming properties and can help soothe the mind and prepare for sleep.
- Offer lemon balm tea or use it in herbal preparations designed to promote peaceful sleep.

4. Passionflower (Passiflora incarnata):

- Passionflower is a calming herb that can help ease anxiety and promote a sense of tranquility before sleep.
- Offer passionflower tea or use it as an ingredient in bedtime herbal blends.

5. Valerian (Valeriana officinalis):

- Valerian is a sedative herb that can promote relaxation and support restful sleep.
- Use valerian root in teas or consider valerian supplements under the guidance of a healthcare professional.

6. Hops (Humulus lupulus):

- Hops is a gentle sedative herb that can help calm the nervous system and promote sleepiness.
- Use hops in teas or incorporate it into herbal preparations for bedtime relaxation.

7. Herbal Pillow Mist:

- Create a soothing herbal pillow mist using a combination of relaxing herbs like lavender, chamomile, and lemon balm.
- Spritz the mist lightly on your child's pillow or bedding before bedtime to create a calming environment.

8. Gentle Massage with Herbal Oils:

- Use a gentle, child-safe herbal oil such as lavender-infused oil to provide a calming massage before bed.
- The rhythmic touch combined with the soothing aroma can help relax your child's body and mind.

Remember to create a consistent bedtime routine and allow enough time for winding down before sleep. Keep the sleep environment comfortable, dark, and quiet to support peaceful sleep.

## 6.3 Supporting Healthy Emotional Well-being in Children

Emotional well-being is essential for children to thrive and navigate the ups and downs of life. Here are strategies and herbal remedies to support healthy emotional well-being in children:

1. Open Communication:

- Encourage open and supportive communication with your child, allowing them to express their emotions and concerns.
- Create a safe space for them to share their thoughts, feelings, and experiences without judgment.

2. Mindfulness and Relaxation:

- Teach your child simple mindfulness and relaxation techniques to help them manage stress and cultivate emotional resilience.
- Breathing exercises, guided visualizations, and gentle yoga can promote a sense of calm and self-awareness.

3. Herbal Mood Lifters:

- Certain herbs have mood-lifting properties and can support emotional well-being.

- St. John's Wort (Hypericum perforatum) and Lemon Balm (Melissa officinalis) are known for their mood-enhancing effects.
- Consult with a healthcare professional or qualified herbalist for appropriate dosages and guidance.

4. Nature Therapy:

- Spending time in nature has a positive impact on emotional well-being.
- Encourage outdoor activities, such as nature walks, gardening, or simply playing in a natural setting, to help your child

connect with nature's calming influence.

5. Emotional Support Herbs:

- Herbs like Rose (Rosa spp.), Linden (Tilia spp.), and Hawthorn (Crataegus spp.) have traditionally been used to support emotional well-being and ease feelings of stress or sadness.
- Incorporate these herbs in teas, herbal blends, or as aromatherapy to provide gentle emotional support.

6. Journaling and Creative Expression:

- Encourage your child to engage in journaling, drawing, or other creative outlets to express their emotions and thoughts.
- Creative expression can help them process their feelings and foster self-reflection.

7. Healthy Lifestyle Habits:

- Support your child's overall well-being by promoting a healthy lifestyle.
- Encourage regular exercise, nutritious meals, adequate sleep, and a balanced routine to support emotional resilience.

8. Seek Professional Support:

- If your child's emotional well-being is significantly impacted or persists over time, seek professional support from a therapist or counselor specializing in child psychology.

Remember that every child is unique, and their emotional well-being may require individualized approaches.

# Chapter 7

# **Enhancing Skin Health and Healing**

## *7.1 Herbal Remedies for Common Skin Issues*

Children often encounter various skin issues, ranging from dryness and irritation to minor cuts and scrapes. Herbal remedies can offer gentle and effective solutions for common skin concerns. Here are some herbal remedies for promoting healthy skin in children:

1. Calendula (Calendula officinalis):

- Calendula is renowned for its soothing and healing properties for the skin.
- Use calendula-infused oil or salve to soothe dry, chapped skin, minor cuts, and irritations.

2. Aloe Vera (Aloe barbadensis):

- Aloe vera has cooling and moisturizing properties that can alleviate sunburns, rashes, and minor skin irritations.
- Apply fresh aloe vera gel directly to the affected area for soothing relief.

3. Chamomile (Matricaria chamomilla):

- Chamomile is known for its anti-inflammatory and calming effects on the skin.
- Prepare a chamomile tea infusion and use it as a gentle wash or compress for irritated or inflamed skin.

4. Lavender (Lavandula angustifolia):

- Lavender has soothing and antiseptic properties, making it useful for minor cuts, burns, and skin irritations.
- Apply diluted lavender essential oil topically or incorporate it into a gentle herbal salve.

5. Plantain (Plantago major):

- Plantain is a common weed with drawing and healing properties for the skin.
- Crush fresh plantain leaves and apply the poultice directly to insect bites, stings, or minor wounds.

6. Comfrey (Symphytum officinale):

- Comfrey contains allantoin, a compound known for promoting cell regeneration and healing of the skin.
- Use comfrey-infused oil or salve to support the healing of minor wounds, cuts, and bruises.

## 7. Tea Tree Oil (Melaleuca alternifolia):

- Tea tree oil possesses antimicrobial properties and can be used sparingly for minor skin infections, acne, or fungal issues.
- Dilute tea tree oil in a carrier oil before applying it to the affected area.

## 8. Herbal Baths:

- Create herbal baths using skin-soothing herbs like oatmeal, chamomile, and calendula.
- Infuse these herbs in warm bathwater and allow your child to soak for gentle relief from skin irritations.

Remember to patch test any herbal remedies before applying them to your child's skin, and discontinue use if any adverse reactions occur. If a skin issue persists or worsens, consult a healthcare professional for further evaluation and guidance.

## 7.2 Nourishing and Soothing Herbal Skin Care

Taking care of your child's skin goes beyond addressing specific issues. Nourishing and soothing herbal skin care practices can promote overall skin health and maintain its natural vitality. Here are some herbal skin care practices to incorporate into your child's routine:

1. Daily Cleansing:

   - Use a gentle herbal cleanser to remove dirt, impurities, and excess oil from your child's skin.
   - Look for cleansers containing herbs like chamomile, lavender, or calendula for their soothing properties.

2. Herbal Toners:

   - Toners help balance the skin's pH levels and tighten pores.
   - Prepare a gentle herbal toner using herbs like rose, witch hazel, or cucumber, and apply it

to your child's skin using a cotton pad.

3. Moisturizing with Herbal Oils:

- Herbal oils can provide deep nourishment and hydration to the skin.
- Choose oils such as jojoba, almond, or rosehip infused with herbs like lavender or chamomile for their soothing properties.
- Apply a small amount of the herbal oil to your child's skin after cleansing or as needed to maintain moisture.

4. Herbal Face Masks:

- Treat your child's skin to a weekly herbal face mask to nourish and rejuvenate.
- Use a blend of powdered herbs like oatmeal, clay, and botanicals suitable for their skin type.
- Mix with water or aloe vera gel to form a paste, apply it to the skin, and leave it on for the recommended time before rinsing off.

5. Herbal Sun Protection:

- Protect your child's skin from the harmful effects of the sun using herbal sunscreens or natural sunblocks.

- Look for products containing herbs like green tea, aloe vera, or raspberry seed oil for their natural sun-protective properties.

6. Herbal Lip Balms:

- Keep your child's lips hydrated and protected with herbal lip balms.
- Look for lip balms containing herbs like calendula, chamomile, or lavender to soothe and moisturize their delicate lips.

7. Herbal Body Care:

- Extend herbal skin care to the whole body by using herbal body washes, lotions, and creams.
- Look for products infused with herbs like chamomile, calendula, or lavender for their soothing and nourishing properties.

Remember to choose herbal skin care products that are specifically formulated for children and free from harsh chemicals or irritants. Perform patch tests before introducing new products and discontinue use if any adverse reactions occur.

## 7.3 Herbal First Aid for Cuts, Scrapes, and Burns

Children are prone to minor cuts, scrapes, and burns as they explore the world around them. Herbal first aid remedies can provide gentle relief and promote healing. Here are some herbal remedies for addressing common minor injuries:

1. Calendula (Calendula officinalis):

   - Calendula is a powerful herb for promoting skin healing and reducing inflammation.
   - Apply a calendula-infused salve or ointment to minor cuts,

scrapes, or burns to accelerate the healing process.

2. Plantain (Plantago major):

- Plantain is known for its drawing and wound-healing properties.
- Create a poultice using crushed fresh plantain leaves and apply it directly to cuts, scrapes, or insect bites.

3. Comfrey (Symphytum officinale):

- Comfrey contains allantoin, a compound that supports cell regeneration and wound healing.
- Use a comfrey-infused oil or salve on minor cuts, scrapes, or

bruises to aid in the healing process.

4. Aloe Vera (Aloe barbadensis):

- Aloe vera has soothing and cooling properties, making it beneficial for minor burns, including sunburns.
- Apply fresh aloe vera gel directly to the affected area for relief and to promote healing.

5. Lavender (Lavandula angustifolia):

- Lavender has antiseptic and calming properties, making it useful for minor cuts, burns, or scrapes.

- Apply diluted lavender essential oil topically or use it in a herbal spray to provide relief and aid in healing.

6. Chamomile (Matricaria chamomilla):

- Chamomile has anti-inflammatory and soothing properties, making it helpful for minor skin irritations and burns.
- Prepare a chamomile tea infusion and use it as a compress or wash for the affected area.

7. Echinacea (Echinacea purpurea):

- Echinacea has antimicrobial and immune-boosting properties that can support wound healing.
- Use echinacea tincture diluted with water as a topical wash for minor cuts or scrapes.

8. Herbal Wound Cleansers:

- Create a gentle herbal wound cleanser using a combination of antimicrobial herbs like lavender, thyme, or tea tree.
- Dilute the herbal tinctures or essential oils in water and use the mixture to cleanse minor wounds before applying other herbal remedies.

Remember to assess the severity of the injury and seek medical attention for deep or serious wounds, severe burns, or any injury requiring professional care.

# Chapter 8

# Herbal Support for Growth and Development

## 8.1 Supporting Healthy Growth with Herbs

Healthy growth and development are crucial for children, and herbs can play a supportive role in promoting overall well-being. Here are some ways herbs can contribute to supporting healthy growth in children:

1. Nourishing Herbal Tonics:

- Herbal tonics can provide essential nutrients to support growth and development.
- Herbs like nettle, alfalfa, and oatstraw are rich in vitamins, minerals, and phytonutrients.
- Create nourishing herbal infusions or incorporate powdered herbs into smoothies or soups for a nutritional boost.

2. Calcium-Rich Herbs:

- Calcium is vital for bone development and growth.
- Incorporate calcium-rich herbs such as horsetail, dandelion greens, and sesame seeds into your child's diet.

- Add these herbs to meals, salads, or herbal teas to support healthy bone growth.

3. Herbal Mineral Support:

- Minerals like zinc, magnesium, and iron are essential for growth and development.
- Incorporate herbs like spirulina, dulse, and chickweed, which are rich in minerals, into your child's diet.
- Consider herbal mineral supplements under the guidance of a healthcare professional or qualified herbalist.

4. Immune-Boosting Herbs:

- A strong immune system is crucial for healthy growth.
- Herbs such as elderberry, astragalus, and echinacea can support immune function in children.
- Prepare immune-boosting herbal teas or incorporate herbal extracts into their daily routine during cold and flu seasons.

5. Digestive Support Herbs:

- Healthy digestion is essential for proper nutrient absorption and growth.

- Herbs like fennel, ginger, and peppermint can aid digestion and alleviate digestive discomfort.
- Use these herbs in herbal teas or incorporate them into meals to support optimal digestion.

6. Adaptogenic Herbs for Stress Management:

- Chronic stress can interfere with growth and development.
- Adaptogenic herbs like ashwagandha, holy basil, and rhodiola can help support the body's stress response.
- Consider using adaptogenic herbs under the guidance of a

healthcare professional or qualified herbalist.

7. Balanced Nutrition:

- Alongside herbal support, provide your child with a balanced and nutrient-dense diet.
- Include a variety of fruits, vegetables, whole grains, and lean proteins to support overall growth and development.

It is important to note that herbs should be used as part of a holistic approach to support healthy growth, and consulting with a healthcare professional or qualified herbalist is recommended to determine appropriate dosages and ensure safety.

## 8.2 Herbal Solutions for Nutritional Needs

Proper nutrition is vital for children's growth, development, and overall health. Alongside a balanced diet, herbs can offer additional support by providing essential nutrients and promoting optimal nutrition. Here are some herbal solutions to address nutritional needs in children:

1. Herbal Infusions and Decoctions:

   - Herbal infusions and decoctions are concentrated forms of herbs that can be used to supplement nutrition.

- Nettle, alfalfa, and red clover are rich in vitamins, minerals, and phytonutrients. Prepare these herbs as infusions or decoctions to enhance nutritional intake.

2. Herbal Powders and Superfoods:

- Incorporate herbal powders and superfoods into your child's diet to provide concentrated nutrition.
- Spirulina, chlorella, moringa, and wheatgrass are nutrient-dense options that can be added to smoothies, yogurt, or baked goods.

3. Herbal Mineral Boosters:

- Minerals are essential for various bodily functions. Certain herbs can provide mineral-rich support.
- Horsetail, dandelion greens, and nettles are herbs known for their high mineral content. Incorporate them into meals or herbal preparations to boost mineral intake.

4. Vitamin-Rich Herbal Teas:

- Herbal teas can be a source of vitamins and antioxidants.
- Rosehip, hibiscus, and lemon balm teas are rich in vitamin C. Enjoy these herbal teas as a refreshing and nutritious beverage.

5. Herbal Calcium Sources:

- Adequate calcium is necessary for strong bones and teeth. Herbs can contribute to calcium intake.
- Include calcium-rich herbs like horsetail, oatstraw, and dandelion greens in your child's diet to support healthy bone development.

6. Herbal Ferments and Probiotics:

- Gut health is crucial for proper nutrient absorption. Herbal ferments and probiotics can promote a healthy digestive system.

- Use herbs like dill, fennel, and ginger to make herbal ferments or incorporate probiotic-rich foods like kefir or sauerkraut into your child's diet.

7. Nutrient-Specific Herbal Supplements:

- In some cases, specific nutrient deficiencies may require targeted herbal supplementation.
- Work with a healthcare professional or qualified herbalist to determine appropriate herbal supplements tailored to your child's nutritional needs.

Remember, herbal solutions should complement a well-rounded and balanced diet, and consulting with a healthcare professional or qualified herbalist is recommended to determine the most suitable herbal approach for your child's nutritional needs.

## 8.3 Boosting Brain Power and Cognitive Function

A child's cognitive development is essential for their learning, memory, and overall brain function. Herbal remedies can play a supportive role in boosting brain power and enhancing cognitive function. Here are some herbal solutions to consider:

1. Rosemary (Rosmarinus officinalis):

- Rosemary is known for its memory-enhancing properties.
- Diffuse rosemary essential oil or incorporate it into massage oils to promote concentration and mental clarity.

2. Ginkgo (Ginkgo biloba):

- Ginkgo is a renowned herb for cognitive support and improving memory.
- Consider using ginkgo supplements or infusing ginkgo leaves to make a tea for cognitive enhancement.

3. Gotu Kola (Centella asiatica):

- Gotu kola is traditionally used to support mental clarity and focus.
- Incorporate gotu kola into herbal teas, tinctures, or capsules to support cognitive function.

4. Bacopa (Bacopa monnieri):

- Bacopa is an herb known for its cognitive-enhancing and memory-improving properties.
- Use bacopa supplements or incorporate dried bacopa leaves into herbal preparations for cognitive support.

5. Lemon Balm (Melissa officinalis):

- Lemon balm has calming and uplifting effects on the nervous system.
- Brew lemon balm tea and offer it to your child to promote a relaxed and focused state of mind.

6. Peppermint (Mentha piperita):

- Peppermint is invigorating and can help stimulate mental alertness.
- Diffuse peppermint essential oil or offer peppermint tea to enhance focus and cognitive function.

7. Brahmi (Bacopa monnieri):

- Brahmi is an Ayurvedic herb known for its ability to support brain function and memory.
- Use brahmi in herbal preparations or consider brahmi supplements under the guidance of a healthcare professional or qualified herbalist.

## 8. Nutrient-Rich Herbal Foods:

- Incorporate nutrient-rich herbs into your child's diet to support brain health.
- Herbs like spinach, turmeric, and sage are known for their brain-boosting properties.

Include them in meals or smoothies.

It's important to note that herbal remedies should be used in conjunction with a healthy diet, regular exercise, and a stimulating environment to support optimal brain development. Additionally, consulting with a healthcare professional or qualified herbalist is recommended, especially when considering herbal supplements.

# Chapter 9

# **Integrating Herbs into Daily Life**

## *9.1 Incorporating Herbs into Meals and Snacks*

Incorporating herbs into meals and snacks is a creative and delicious way to enhance flavor, provide nutritional benefits, and introduce children to the world of herbal cuisine. Here are some ideas for incorporating herbs into your child's meals and snacks:

1. Herb-infused Oils and Vinegars:

- Create herb-infused oils or vinegars by steeping herbs like basil, thyme, or rosemary in quality oils or vinegars.
- Use these infused oils or vinegars in salad dressings, marinades, or drizzle them over roasted vegetables for added flavor.

2. Fresh Herb Toppings:

- Sprinkle freshly chopped herbs such as parsley, cilantro, or chives on top of soups, stews, salads, or pasta dishes.
- The vibrant colors and fragrant aromas of fresh herbs will not

only enhance the visual appeal but also add a burst of flavor.

3. Herbal Butters and Spreads:

- Blend softened butter or cream cheese with chopped herbs like dill, basil, or tarragon to create herb-infused spreads.
- Spread these flavored butters or cream cheeses on toast, crackers, or use them as a tasty addition to sandwiches.

4. Herbal Smoothies and Juices:

- Add fresh herbs like mint, basil, or parsley to smoothies or freshly squeezed juices.
- The herbs will infuse the beverages with refreshing flavors

and provide additional nutritional benefits.

5. Herb-infused Water and Herbal Iced Teas:

- Infuse water with herbs such as cucumber and mint or lemon and thyme for a refreshing and flavorful drink.
- Brew herbal iced teas using herbs like chamomile, hibiscus, or lavender, sweeten if desired, and serve over ice.

6. Herbal Seasoning Blends:

- Create custom herbal seasoning blends by combining dried herbs like oregano, thyme, and garlic powder.

- Use these blends to season meats, poultry, fish, roasted vegetables, or sprinkle them over popcorn for a flavorful snack.

7. Herbal Baked Goods:

- Experiment with herbs in baked goods by adding them to bread, muffins, cookies, or cakes.
- Herbs like lavender, rosemary, or lemon balm can add unique flavors and aromas to sweet treats.

8. Herbal Infused Honey or Syrups:

- Infuse honey or syrups with herbs like ginger, cinnamon, or lavender for a sweet and herbal twist.
- Drizzle these infused sweeteners over pancakes, waffles, yogurt, or fruit for a delightful treat.

Remember to consider your child's preferences and any allergies or sensitivities when incorporating herbs into their meals and snacks. Start with milder herbs and gradually introduce stronger flavors. Encourage your child to explore and appreciate the diverse tastes and aromas that herbs bring to their meals.

## 9.2 Herbal Teas, Infusions, and Tonics for Kids

Herbal teas, infusions, and tonics can be a delightful and nourishing way to introduce children to the world of herbs. These beverages offer a wide range of flavors, aromas, and health benefits. Here are some herbal options specifically tailored for kids:

1. Fruity Herbal Iced Teas:

   - Prepare refreshing herbal iced teas using fruity herbs like hibiscus, rosehips, or lemon verbena.
   - Sweeten with a natural sweetener like honey or a touch of fruit

juice for a delicious and hydrating beverage.

2. Calming Herbal Infusions:

- Create soothing herbal infusions using herbs such as chamomile, lemon balm, or lavender.
- These infusions can be enjoyed warm or chilled and are ideal for promoting relaxation and a sense of calm.

3. Immune-Boosting Herbal Tonics:

- Support your child's immune system with herbal tonics made from immune-boosting herbs like elderberry, echinacea, or astragalus.

- Combine these herbs with a bit of honey or lemon juice for added flavor and immune support.

4. Digestive Herbal Teas:

- Promote healthy digestion with herbal teas containing digestive-supporting herbs like peppermint, fennel, or ginger.
- These teas can provide relief from digestive discomfort and are especially beneficial after meals.

5. Energy-Boosting Herbal Blends:

- Create energizing herbal blends using herbs like ginseng, ginkgo, or rosemary to provide a natural pick-me-up.
- These blends can be enjoyed as warm teas or iced for a refreshing energy boost.

6. Nourishing Herbal Infusions:

- Nettle, oatstraw, and red clover are herbs rich in vitamins and minerals.
- Prepare nourishing herbal infusions by steeping these herbs in hot water for an extended period to extract their beneficial nutrients.

7. Minty Herbal Refreshers:

- Mint herbs like spearmint or peppermint make invigorating and refreshing herbal teas.
- Serve these teas chilled with a squeeze of lemon for a cooling and revitalizing beverage.

8. Herbal Lemonades:

- Combine freshly squeezed lemon juice with herbal infusions or teas for a zesty and herbal twist on traditional lemonade.
- Experiment with herbs like lemongrass, lemon verbena, or lemon balm to add unique flavors.

When preparing herbal beverages for children, it's important to consider their preferences, any allergies, and sensitivities. Start with milder flavors and gradually introduce stronger herbal profiles. You can also involve your child in the preparation process, allowing them to select herbs and create their own herbal concoctions.

Remember to consult with a healthcare professional or qualified herbalist if your child has any specific health conditions or if you have concerns about potential herb-drug interactions.

## 9.3 Herbal Bathing and Body Care Rituals

Herbal bathing and body care rituals offer a soothing and rejuvenating experience for children while providing numerous benefits for their skin, relaxation, and overall well-being. Here are some herbal bathing and body care ideas to incorporate into your child's routine:

1. Herbal Bath Infusions:

   - Create herbal bath infusions by steeping herbs like chamomile, lavender, or calendula in warm water.

- Strain the herbs and add the infused water to your child's bath for a calming and aromatic soak.

2. Herbal Bath Bags:

- Make herbal bath bags by filling muslin or cotton bags with a mixture of herbs like oatmeal, lavender, or rose petals.
- Hang these bags under the faucet while filling the bath to allow the water to flow through them, releasing the herbal goodness.

3. Herb-Infused Bath Oils:

- Infuse carrier oils like sweet almond or jojoba oil with herbs such as rosemary, chamomile, or calendula.

- Add a few drops of the infused oil to your child's bathwater to moisturize and nourish their skin.

4. Soothing Herbal Bath Salts:

- Combine Epsom salt or sea salt with dried herbs like lavender, chamomile, or rosemary.
- Add a small amount of the herbal bath salts to your child's bath to promote relaxation and ease muscle tension.

5. Herbal Hair Rinse:

- Create an herbal hair rinse by steeping herbs like rosemary, nettle, or chamomile in hot water.
- After shampooing, pour the herbal infusion over your child's hair as a final rinse for added shine and scalp health.

6. Herbal Body Scrubs:

- Prepare gentle herbal body scrubs using ingredients like sugar, salt, or oatmeal combined with herbs such as lavender, chamomile, or calendula.
- Gently massage the scrub onto your child's skin during bath time to exfoliate and leave their skin feeling soft and smooth.

7. Aromatherapy Bath Bombs:

- Create aromatic bath bombs using essential oils with calming properties, such as lavender or chamomile.
- Drop a bath bomb into your child's bathwater, and let them enjoy the relaxing scents and fizzing experience.

8. Herbal Moisturizers:

- Use herbal-infused oils or herbal extracts to create homemade moisturizers for your child's skin.
- Calendula, chamomile, and lavender are herbs known for

their soothing and nourishing properties.

Always ensure the safety and suitability of herbs and essential oils for your child's age and any known allergies or sensitivities. It's recommended to perform a patch test and dilute essential oils properly before use.

By incorporating herbal bathing and body care rituals into your child's routine, you can create a nurturing and sensory experience that promotes relaxation, skin health, and overall well-being.

# Chapter 10

# Holistic Approaches to Children's Health

## 10.1 Combining Herbs with Mind-Body Practices

Combining herbs with mind-body practices can create a powerful synergy that promotes holistic well-being for children. These practices help cultivate mindfulness, relaxation, and self-awareness while incorporating the therapeutic benefits of herbs. Here are some ways to combine herbs with mind-body practices for your child:

1. Herbal Aromatherapy:

   - Incorporate herbs with calming scents, such as lavender, chamomile, or lemon balm, into aromatherapy practices.
   - Diffuse essential oils or create herbal sachets for your child to inhale during meditation, yoga, or relaxation exercises.

2. Herbal Meditation and Visualization:

   - Create a peaceful and serene environment for your child's meditation practice using herbs like sage, frankincense, or sandalwood.

- Burn dried herbs or use essential oils in a diffuser to enhance the ambiance and create a calming atmosphere.

3. Herbal Mindfulness Exercises:

- Introduce your child to mindfulness exercises while engaging with herbs.
- Encourage them to explore the colors, textures, and scents of herbs, bringing their full attention to the present moment.

4. Herbal Yoga and Stretching:

- Incorporate herbs into your child's yoga or stretching routines to enhance the mind-body connection.

- Diffuse calming herbs, apply herbal-infused oils to their body, or use herbal eye pillows during relaxation poses.

5. Herbal Tea Ceremonies:

- Create a mindful tea-drinking ritual with your child using herbal teas.
- Encourage them to savor each sip, noticing the flavors, aromas, and sensations that arise, fostering a sense of presence.

6. Herbal Breathing Exercises:

- Combine breathing exercises with the aromas of calming herbs to promote relaxation and grounding.
- Inhale the soothing scents of herbs while practicing deep breathing or guided breathing exercises with your child.

7. Herbal Journaling:

- Encourage your child to keep an herbal journal where they can record their experiences, thoughts, and feelings related to herbs.
- This practice fosters self-reflection, mindfulness, and

a deeper connection to the natural world.

8. Herbal Self-Care Rituals:

- Teach your child the importance of self-care through herbal-infused baths, massages, or foot soaks.
- Guide them in applying herbal oils or lotions to their body while emphasizing the intention of self-nurturing and relaxation.

Remember to tailor these practices to your child's age and interests, making them enjoyable and accessible. Always ensure the safety and suitability of herbs and essential oils for your child, following proper dilution guidelines and consulting with a healthcare professional if needed.


## 10.2 Nature's Healing Power: Outdoor Activities and Herb Exploration

Spending time in nature and exploring the world of herbs outdoors can provide a wealth of healing experiences for children. Engaging in outdoor activities and herb exploration not only promotes physical activity but also fosters a deeper connection with the natural world. Here are some ideas to combine nature and herb exploration for your child:

1. Herb Walks and Nature Hikes:

- Take your child on herb walks and nature hikes to explore different environments and discover herbs growing in the wild.
- Encourage them to observe, touch, and smell the herbs while learning about their properties and traditional uses.

2. Herb Identification and Plant Pressing:

- Teach your child how to identify different herbs using field guides or smartphone apps.
- Collect small samples of herbs and press them between the pages of a book to create a herb collection for future reference.

3. Herb Gardening:

- Involve your child in planting and maintaining a herb garden at home or in a community garden.
- Let them experience the joy of watching herbs grow, tending to them, and eventually harvesting and using them for various purposes.

4. Herb Crafts and Art:

- Encourage your child to express their creativity by incorporating herbs into crafts and art projects.
- They can make herbal wreaths, create herbal-infused playdough,

or paint with herbal pigments made from plants like turmeric or beetroot.

5. Herb Scavenger Hunts:

- Organize herb-themed scavenger hunts where your child can search for specific herbs or natural objects associated with herbs, such as leaves, flowers, or seeds.
- This activity helps develop their observational skills while deepening their knowledge of herbs.

6. Herb-Inspired Picnics:

- Plan outdoor picnics and include herbal treats and snacks made with fresh herbs.
- Your child can experience the flavors and aromas of herbs in a natural setting, connecting their senses with the surrounding environment.

7. Herbal Crafting and DIY Projects:

- Engage your child in hands-on herbal crafting projects, such as making herbal sachets, herbal bath bombs, or herbal dream pillows.
- These activities allow them to explore the practical and creative aspects of working with herbs.

8. Mindful Nature Meditation:

- Find a quiet spot in nature where your child can practice mindful meditation surrounded by the sights, sounds, and scents of herbs and the natural world.
- Guide them through simple breathing exercises and encourage them to connect with the grounding energy of the earth.

Remember to prioritize safety during outdoor activities by applying appropriate sun protection, using insect repellents when necessary, and being aware of any potential hazards in the environment. Teach your child about ethical foraging practices, respecting plant habitats, and the importance of sustainability.

## 10.3 Cultivating a Healthy Lifestyle for Children

Cultivating a healthy lifestyle is essential for children's overall well-being, and it goes beyond just incorporating herbs into their routine. It involves creating a balanced and nurturing environment that supports their physical, mental, and emotional health. Here are some key areas to focus on when cultivating a healthy lifestyle for children:

1. Nutritious Diet:

- Provide a well-rounded and nutritious diet that includes a variety of fruits, vegetables, whole grains, lean proteins, and healthy fats.
- Encourage your child to eat mindfully, emphasizing the importance of listening to their body's hunger and fullness cues.

2. Regular Physical Activity:

- Encourage your child to engage in regular physical activity that they enjoy, such as sports, dancing, cycling, or simply playing outdoors.
- Aim for at least 60 minutes of moderate to vigorous physical

activity per day to promote physical fitness and overall health.

3. Adequate Sleep:

- Establish consistent bedtime routines and ensure that your child gets enough sleep according to their age.
- Create a calm and soothing sleep environment, free from electronic devices, to support restful and rejuvenating sleep.

4. Emotional Well-being:

- Foster emotional well-being by creating a supportive and

nurturing environment where your child feels loved, valued, and understood.

- Encourage open communication, active listening, and provide guidance and coping strategies for managing emotions.

5. Mindful Technology Use:

- Promote healthy technology habits by setting limits on screen time and encouraging your child to engage in other activities, such as reading, playing, or pursuing hobbies.
- Encourage mindful technology use by discussing the importance of balancing screen time with

outdoor play and social interactions.

6. Hygiene and Self-care:

- Teach your child about good hygiene practices, including regular handwashing, dental care, and personal grooming.
- Encourage self-care activities such as bathing, brushing teeth, and caring for their skin, emphasizing the importance of taking care of their bodies.

7. Positive Social Connections:

- Encourage your child to build positive and supportive

relationships with peers, family, and community.

- Foster opportunities for social interactions through playdates, extracurricular activities, and community involvement.

8. Time in Nature:

- Prioritize spending time in nature as a family, engaging in outdoor activities, and appreciating the natural world.
- Nature provides numerous benefits for children's physical and mental health, fostering a sense of wonder, curiosity, and connection.

Remember, cultivating a healthy lifestyle is a gradual process that requires consistency, patience, and flexibility. Lead by example and involve your child in decision-making processes related to their health. Encourage them to develop autonomy and make choices that align with their well-being.

By focusing on these aspects and creating a nurturing environment, you can cultivate a healthy lifestyle that supports your child's growth, development, and overall well-being. This holistic approach will lay the foundation for a lifetime of good health habits and a positive relationship with their body, mind, and the world around them.

# Conclusion

## <u>Empowering Parents as Herb Doctors for Their Children</u>

In today's fast-paced world, parents play a vital role in ensuring the health and well-being of their children. By embracing the power of herbs and natural remedies, parents can become the herb doctors for their children, empowering themselves with knowledge and practical skills to support their children's health.

Through this comprehensive guide, we have explored the fascinating world of herbs for children's health. From understanding the history and traditions of herbal healing to learning about the benefits, precautions, and dosage guidelines, we have covered a wide range of topics. We have delved into various aspects of children's health, including immune support, digestive wellness, respiratory health, emotional well-being, skincare, and more.

By incorporating herbs into our children's lives, we tap into the bountiful gifts of nature. Herbs offer a gentle and holistic approach to health, providing natural solutions that align with our body's innate healing abilities. They can complement conventional treatments and empower parents to take a proactive role in their children's well-being.

As herb doctors for our children, we have explored various herbal preparations, sourcing and growing herbs, and using tools and supplies effectively. We have learned about the importance of safety considerations, dosage guidelines, and the significance of consulting healthcare professionals when needed.

Furthermore, we have seen how herbs can be integrated into everyday life, from meals and snacks to teas, infusions, and tonics. We have explored the benefits of outdoor activities, herb exploration, and connecting with nature to enhance the healing experience. By combining herbs with mind-body practices, we create a harmonious integration of the natural world and inner well-being for our children.

Throughout this journey, we have emphasized the importance of a holistic approach to children's health. We have recognized the significance of a nutritious diet, regular physical activity, adequate sleep, emotional well-being, and positive social connections. By cultivating a healthy lifestyle, we create a strong foundation for our children's overall well-being.

As we conclude this guide, let us remember that being an herb doctor for our children is an ongoing learning process. It requires curiosity, open-mindedness, and a willingness to adapt to the unique needs of each child. It is through our love, dedication, and commitment that we can nurture our children's health and help them thrive.

So, let us embrace the power of herbs, embrace our role as herb doctors, and embark on this journey with confidence and compassion. Together, we can create a healthier, happier future for our children—one herb at a time.

# Appendix

## Quick Reference Guide to Essential Herbs and Remedies

In this appendix, you will find a quick reference guide to essential herbs and remedies discussed throughout the book. This guide serves as a handy resource for parents, providing a summary of key herbs and their associated benefits for children's health.

1. Chamomile (Matricaria chamomilla):

    - Benefits: Calming, promotes relaxation, supports digestive health, soothes skin irritations, aids in sleep.

225

- Forms: Tea, herbal infusion, tincture, bath.

2. Echinacea (Echinacea purpurea):

  - Benefits: Boosts immune system, supports respiratory health, helps fight common colds and infections.
  - Forms: Tincture, capsules, herbal tea.

3. Ginger (Zingiber officinale):

  - Benefits: Aids digestion, relieves nausea and vomiting, supports immune function, reduces inflammation.

- Forms: Fresh ginger root, powdered ginger, ginger tea.

4. Lemon Balm (Melissa officinalis):

- Benefits: Calms anxiety and stress, promotes relaxation, aids digestion, supports restful sleep.
- Forms: Tea, herbal infusion, tincture, essential oil.

5. Peppermint (Mentha piperita):

- Benefits: Relieves digestive discomfort, eases headaches, soothes respiratory congestion, freshens breath.
- Forms: Tea, herbal infusion, essential oil (topical use).

6. Calendula (Calendula officinalis):

- Benefits: Soothes skin irritations, promotes wound healing, reduces inflammation, supports healthy skin.
- Forms: Infused oil, salve, cream, herbal tea (external use).

7. Elderberry (Sambucus nigra):

- Benefits: Boosts immune system, helps prevent and treat cold and flu symptoms, rich in antioxidants.
- Forms: Syrup, capsules, herbal tea.

8. Lavender (Lavandula angustifolia):

- Benefits: Calming and relaxing, promotes sleep, relieves anxiety and stress, soothes skin irritations.
- Forms: Essential oil (aromatherapy, topical use), herbal infusion.

9. Marshmallow Root (Althaea officinalis):

- Benefits: Soothes irritated mucous membranes, supports respiratory health, aids digestion.
- Forms: Tea, herbal infusion, powdered root (external use).

10.   Oatstraw (Avena sativa):

- Benefits: Nourishes the nervous system, promotes relaxation, supports healthy skin, aids digestion.
- Forms: Tea, herbal infusion.

11.   Catnip (Nepeta cataria):

- Benefits: Calming and soothing, relieves restlessness, aids in digestion, supports healthy sleep.
- Forms: Tea, herbal infusion, tincture.

12.   Dandelion (Taraxacum officinale):

- Benefits: Supports liver health, aids in detoxification, promotes healthy digestion, rich in vitamins and minerals.
- Forms: Herbal infusion, tincture, roasted dandelion root tea.

13.  Hawthorn (Crataegus spp.):

- Benefits: Supports cardiovascular health, promotes healthy blood circulation, helps regulate blood pressure.
- Forms: Tincture, capsules, herbal tea.

14.  Mullein (Verbascum thapsus):

- Benefits: Soothes respiratory issues, relieves coughs and congestion, supports healthy lung function.
- Forms: Herbal infusion, tincture, respiratory steam.

15. Nettle (Urtica dioica):

- Benefits: Nourishes the body with essential nutrients, supports healthy immune function, promotes healthy skin.
- Forms: Tea, herbal infusion, capsules.

16. Plantain (Plantago spp.):

- Benefits: Soothes skin irritations, promotes wound healing, relieves insect bites and stings.
- Forms: Poultice, infused oil, salve.

17.   Rosehip (Rosa spp.):

- Benefits: Rich in vitamin C and antioxidants, supports immune health, promotes healthy skin.
- Forms: Herbal infusion, syrup, capsules.

18.   Skullcap (Scutellaria lateriflora):

- Benefits: Calms nervous tension and anxiety, promotes relaxation, supports healthy sleep.

- Forms: Tincture, herbal infusion.

19.  Thyme (Thymus vulgaris):

- Benefits: Supports respiratory health, relieves coughs and congestion, has antimicrobial properties.
- Forms: Herbal infusion, essential oil (topical use), culinary use.

20.  Yarrow (Achillea millefolium):

- Benefits: Promotes wound healing, supports healthy digestion, has anti-inflammatory properties.
- Forms: Herbal infusion, tincture, topical use (powder or salve).

Remember to research each herb thoroughly, follow proper dosage guidelines, and consult with a healthcare professional or herbalist for personalized advice. Additionally, ensure that the herbs you choose are sourced from reputable suppliers and are safe for your child's age and health condition.

By expanding your knowledge of these essential herbs and remedies, you can further enhance your ability to provide natural support for your child's health and well-being.

# Glossary

## **Key Terms and Definitions**

Here is a glossary of key terms and definitions related to herbs and children's health, providing clarity and understanding of important concepts discussed in this book:

1. Herbal Medicine: The use of plants and plant extracts for medicinal purposes, aimed at promoting health and treating various ailments.

2. Infusion: A method of extracting the beneficial properties of herbs by steeping them in hot water for a period of time, similar to making tea.

3. Tincture: A concentrated herbal extract obtained by soaking herbs in alcohol or a mixture of alcohol and water, often used for its therapeutic effects.

4. Dosage: The specific amount of a herbal remedy recommended for use, taking into consideration factors such as age, weight, and health condition.

5. Holistic Health: A comprehensive approach to health that considers the physical, mental, emotional, and spiritual well-being of an individual.

6. Immune System: The body's defense mechanism against pathogens, viruses, and other foreign substances,

responsible for protecting overall health and fighting infections.

7. Digestive Health: The optimal functioning of the digestive system, including the processes of digestion, absorption, and elimination.

8. Respiratory Health: The well-being of the respiratory system, which includes the lungs, bronchi, trachea, and other related structures involved in breathing and oxygen exchange.

9. Emotional Well-being: The state of emotional balance and mental wellness, encompassing one's emotional intelligence, coping skills, and overall emotional health.

10. Skin Care: Practices and products used to maintain the health, appearance, and integrity of the skin, which is the body's largest organ.

11. Mind-Body Practices: Techniques that integrate the mind and body to promote holistic well-being, such as meditation, yoga, mindfulness, and breathing exercises.

12. Nutritional Needs: The specific dietary requirements necessary for optimal growth, development, and overall health, including the intake of essential nutrients.

13. Cognitive Function: The mental processes and abilities related to acquiring knowledge, memory, attention, perception, problem-solving, and decision-making.

14. Aromatherapy: The therapeutic use of aromatic plant extracts, such as essential oils, to promote physical, emotional, and mental well-being.

15. Outdoor Activities: Recreational and educational pursuits that take place in natural environments, promoting physical activity, connection with nature, and overall well-being.

16. Detoxification: The process of eliminating toxins and waste products

from the body, often through the liver, kidneys, lymphatic system, and sweat glands.

17. Antioxidants: Substances that help protect the body's cells from damage caused by free radicals, which are unstable molecules that can contribute to various diseases and aging.

18. Nervous System: The complex network of nerves and cells that transmit signals between different parts of the body, responsible for regulating bodily functions and coordinating responses.

19. Herbal Infusion: An herbal tea made by steeping herbs in hot water for a

certain period, allowing the water to extract the medicinal properties of the herbs.

20.   Poultice: A soft, moist mass of herbs or other substances applied to the skin to relieve inflammation, soothe wounds, or draw out toxins.

This glossary provides a foundation for understanding the terminology used throughout the book, enabling readers to navigate the content with ease and clarity.